The Caregiver –
The Second Cancer Patient
Making Better Lemonade

by James S. Liao

Foreword

I would like to thank Jane Wilkins Michael whose upcoming book, <u>Better Than Before</u>, assisted me in dealing with the passing of my wife.

I hope that my book will assist others in dealing with the illness of a loved one, especially if one becomes the primary non-medical caregiver.

The photo on the cover of this book is of my Jeep. I struggled for a long time to find a photo that I thought would be appropriate. But as I recently sold my Jeep, it occurred to me that this car was the vehicle I used to take my wife to various medical appointments. It was the car that I depended upon not to fail and always be reliable – in some ways an extension of the role and responsibility of the caregiver.

Musee Des Beaux Arts
by W.H. Auden

About suffering they were never wrong,
The Old Masters; how well, they understood
Its human position; how it takes place
While someone else is eating or opening a window or just walking dully along;
How, when the aged are reverently, passionately waiting
For the miraculous birth, there always must be
Children who did not specially want it to happen, skating
On a pond at the edge of the wood:
They never forgot
That even the dreadful martyrdom must run its course
Anyhow in a corner, some untidy spot
Where the dogs go on with their doggy life and the torturer's horse
Scratches its innocent behind on a tree.
In Breughel's Icarus, for instance: how everything turns away
Quite leisurely from the disaster; the ploughman may
Have heard the splash, the forsaken cry,
But for him it was not an important failure; the sun shone
As it had to on the white legs disappearing into the green
Water; and the expensive delicate ship that must have seen
Something amazing, a boy falling out of the sky,
had somewhere to get to and sailed calmly on.

Table of Contents

Chapter 1 - Why *Musee Des Beaux Arts*?

We all tend to view ourselves to a greater or lesser degree as the center of our own universe and that what is happening to us is the most important thing that we (and everyone else) "should" care about. The reality is: we are not at the center of the universe and even our closest friends and loved ones do go about their own business. They have to. It is not a negative statement about how insensitive or unfeeling they are. It is human nature.

Even the medical professionals will have a degree of detachment – remember, you are not the only case on which they are working. They may be your physician (and their staff), but they are not your *private* physician.

Even the primary caregiver cannot sacrifice him or herself totally to the patient, to the exclusion of taking care of themselves.

So, we must be prepared to be ignored to one degree or another, by our friends and loved ones from time to time, just as Icarus was, despite his most unusual circumstances.

Chapter 2 - When It First Happens

When the patient first learns of the news of the diagnosis, a second patient – the caregiver is also created. That person (the second patient) may not know it at the time (as in many cases when the process starts), but one person eventually emerges as the "go-to" person, the one that can be relied upon, or the one that has no choice but to be the one to be relied upon.

The first patient will experience varying levels of anger, guilt, self pity, fear. You name it, the first patient, even if not expressed verbally or outwardly, will experience these and other emotional highs and lows.

If you understand that you are, or have become, the primary *non-medical* caregiver, you are forced to deal with two people's emotional and psychological issues – the patient's and yours. But, the added difficulty is that you must deal with the patient's emotions and feelings before you can deal with your own. This will be more difficult, bluntly, if you, as the caregiver, are unable to be the "Rock of Gibraltar".

Yes, I have read articles and heard social services professionals talk about how the caregiver should also express or vent their emotions, even with the patient. But I only agree in part. The patient needs the reassurance, support and strength of someone else – that is YOU. If you cannot be that person, you should think seriously about letting someone else be the primary caregiver.

I cried, emoted and felt all the negative emotions as did my wife, but I never wanted to express those negative feelings in front of her – she already felt bad for herself and she would have felt worse if she believed that her illness had made me suffer too.

The oncologists and their staff all spoke about maintaining a positive attitude as part of the treatment process, in addition to the radiation and chemotherapy. The will to fight, to go on and to endure the illness and the side effects of the treatment can only be achieved in a positive atmosphere. If either the patient or caregiver does not believe in success, there will be failure.

Dealing with two people's emotional states will be difficult. As noted in the foreword, having read a draft of my friend's book, <u>Better Than Before</u>, gave me a better sense of what my wife and I were about to go through emotionally and spiritually. As the caregiver, you will be pushed to your physical, mental, emotional and spiritual limits in your role. The biggest toll on me was when my wife directed her anger and frustration at me. This is what happens to caregivers. They become the brunt of all the fear, anger, pain and frustration of being ill and being subjected to humbling or undignified situations in the course of treatment and at various medical facilities, no matter how great, modern or best in class. I had to hold it all in and not lash back because I knew she was hurting and needed me to be the only one to whom she could "let it all hang out".

But, my book is not mainly about how to deal with the emotional and spiritual issues of the caregiver. First, I was raised with traditional male expectations of being stoic. Second, I'm not by nature an extrovert. Third, I'm not trained to be a social worker.

I can only speak from my personal experiences, thinking that I managed to keep our lives under control. In looking back, I found ways of organizing and disciplining my actions that I thought allowed me to give my wife the maximum amount of care that I could. I hope that some of the methods I used will help someone else in the same situation as I found myself – The Caregiver – the Second Cancer Patient.

Chapter 3 - The Second Patient - the Caregiver

This will be my only "preachy" part of the book. I'm sure you're familiar with the concept (and I'll paraphrase) that when life gives you lemons, make lemonade. My corollary is to maker better lemonade.

Bad things will happen to all of us. We are not being punished by some deity or force for having done evil things. Bad things happen to good people. Good people can become *better* people, better lemonade from these adversities.

Lemons are bitter or sour, depending on your taste. We have a choice: you can let the taste make you bitter and sour. Or, as in cooking, you can choose to use this bitter/sour contrast to enhance and let us enjoy the sweet and savory tastes more. I prefer to allow it to help me taste and enjoy the happy moments of life more - better.

Chapter 4 - How I Learned to be a Caregiver

- Take care of the patient like a child growing in reverse
- You must also do so many other things not related to direct patient care
- Know when you need and seek out help

Take care of the patient like a child growing in reverse

This may sound offensive to some to treat the patient, your loved one, as more and more of a child, but you have to be prepared to *progressively* do this as the effects of the illness and the treatment proceeds.

Maybe another analogy is the scene from the movie, "2001 A Space Odyssey", where the protagonist, astronaut, David Bowman (played by Keir Dullea), begins to remove the memory cards of HAL, the computer. At first, HAL still seems to be functioning normally, but slowly, HAL begins to falter until the last card is removed.

In the beginning, as the chemo treatment began, I noticed that my wife who was astute with numbers (as she was a career banker) started to have little lapses of memory or inability to perform relatively simple mathematical tasks. She also began to lose her ability to multi-task, or switch from one task to another mentally. As she had brain tumors, these symptoms were most likely a result of both the illness and the side effects of the treatment.

It was hard and a shock for me to see a person who had accomplished skills begin to falter at performing those skills. I had to make adjustments of how to interact with her, reminding myself that her forgetfulness or difficulty in performing certain tasks were now part of the new reality of our relationship AND NOT HER FAULT.

After a couple of months, the decline in her abilities ceased. It appeared that the tumors had stopped growing. While her abilities did not improve, her performance level remained steady. This allowed us to establish a daily, weekly and monthly routine for both of us. She could walk, drive, work and be by herself without any issues. This seemed a success for her (and the oncologists agreed and were optimistic). If this condition remained stable at this level, I never would have written this book as our lives had only been somewhat negatively impacted.

But after eight months, the MRI showed a new tumor, and then a month later, another tumor. It was then that the chemo was changed a few times (to no avail) and she began to lose use of her left leg, as one of the new tumors was affecting her left side motor skills. Ultimately, she lost the ability to control and use both her left leg and left arm. The progression of this loss of use, looking back, was very quick – only a few months. But for both of us living with this hour by hour, day by day, it seemed to be a slow, interminable grind of anger, pain, despair and, fear for both of us – to suffer and to watch someone suffer.

The rapid rate of her decline made the "earth constantly shift underneath me". As I was responding to one level of decline and adjusting my schedule, shifting furniture around, purchasing medical accessories, within approximately two weeks, her condition worsened so that my earlier efforts and expenditures were for naught.

This is how I came to the *modus operandi* of looking upon her as a child who was not growing and becoming more independent, but just the reverse. At first, she could feed herself, but then, I had to assist and eventually, had to spoon feed her. But unlike a child, she understood and was scared by her declining condition.

My point simply is that you have to be prepared for the patient to become more and more dependent as the illness progresses – more dependent on the caregiver to take care of two physical bodies.

You must also do so many other things too not related to direct patient care

If having to perform physical tasks for two persons wasn't difficult enough, the caregiver has to take on the all the other chores and activities that the patient did, in her/his pre-illness condition. As most modern couples do, we split the household chores tailored or adapted to our likes and dislikes, or by relative convenience of one person to perform that task. Now, the caregiver must do all the tasks, or find someone to assist to do certain tasks. As we did not have children, nor did we have maids or cooks, we did everything ourselves.

And to further add to the burden of the caregiver, I was beginning to realize that my wife was entering her final phase of life – very quickly. Now, I had to begin to think about all the legal, insurance, tax, final arrangements and family affairs that would needed to be addressed. All this while my wife needed visits to the emergency room, stays in the hospital and rehabilitation facilities and I was constantly purchasing new medical accessories trying to make her life easier.

Yes, I began to burn out – physically, psychologically and emotionally.

Know when you need and seek out help

It has been said that one of the most difficult things in life is to know oneself. It is hoped that as one proceeds in life and encounters good and bad situations, one can learn more about oneself.

I think that I was not sure when I needed others to help. But it was after one round of stay at the hospital that the discharge planner, knowing my wife's declining condition, suggested that one of the visiting nurse organizations be contacted to come and assist us upon her return home.

I think I can only say that I "felt" that more was needed, but I didn't know what that "more" was. But, I was willing to listen when I knew needed help. I URGE YOU TO LISTEN AND BE RECEPTIVE to professionals who have much more experience than we have in these matters.

The next several chapters deal with some of the day to day tools or "tricks" I learned to use to help me be as efficient as I could in being a caregiver. There are no secret things to do or secret ways of doing things. Some of them will seem totally obvious, but when you're under stress, your mind does not always function at full ability. If you can accept that your mental performance will also be negatively affected as the level of stress increases for the caregiver, then you can accept considering the use of these simple, but effective ways to get through the task of being a good caregiver.

Chapter 5 - Use the Internet - Learn all you can about the cancer

While there are cautionary stories about not relying on Internet sources as being accurate, I will say that learning about the specific cancer on the Internet is a great way to understand something about how the illness is going to affect the patient and, then affect the caregiver.

Doing a simple keyword search will bring up many useful links. Many of the links will have the same information, but occasionally one will provide additional data.

Having read these sites, I felt better prepared to interact with the medical profession. I knew about the "buzz words" they were using. If what they said seemed to contradict what I thought I read online, I felt more confident in questioning them on the aspect that had the contradiction. Often, the more intelligent questions you can ask, the more information the oncologists or their staff will provide. They're not being secretive; they have other patients and they're trying to be efficient for all their patients. But if you do ask them, they will take the time and will willingly answer them.

If there was anything new that was mentioned to us or, if some aspect was more emphasized which I had only looked at in passing, I would go back on the Internet and do research.

This is a repetitive process of getting new information, asking questions and doing more independent research.

Chapter 6 – Learning to listen – what was said and what was not

The caregiver needs to be the patient advocate, be a second set of ears. The patient has so much swirling around in his/her mind that it should not be surprising that they misheard some statement or instruction.

My wife and I each took separate notes when meeting with the oncologists. As there would be a fair amount of time between meetings, we would compare notes to see if what I heard was the same as what she had. If there was any difference, when the meeting resumed, we went over those points again. As we generally took the train into the city for her treatments and meetings, on the way home, we would again compare notes.

As I noted earlier, the entire medical staff was very willing to repeat anything that was previously discussed. They understand the people under duress can misinterpret comments and they, too, have every desire and incentive to convey the right information.

One area which was key was the pharmaceutical instructions – how often, with or without food, before or after dinner, before she went to bed or just after she woke up. Given how many prescriptions can be given to you, and learning the actual and brand names of the drugs can be disconcerting and confusing. The medical staff always tries to be helpful, but when you get home, you have to be clear yourselves about how to take the medicine.

She began to use a magic marker to mark up the bottles with her shorthand so that she would know how to refer to the different medications. I adopted her shorthand in daily conversation and that helped the communication process.

But in our various meetings and taking notes, it was clear that sometimes a direct question was not answered. The art of listening is twofold: (1) knowing what was actually said, as opposed to being implied and, (2) knowing what was not said. Sometimes, watching or reading the text of a politician trying to squirm their way out of an embarrassing situation is a good way of teaching yourself how to really listen.

It was the few times when the oncologist would deflect or partially answer a question that I paid more attention. What did he really, actually say? And, why would he not answer the question directly? Maybe the question did not make sense to the oncologist in his medical context and experience. I would try to rephrase the question and note the answer and compare it to the previous answer. These were more often than not the times when my wife and I would have differences in our notes – she was hearing one thing as the patient and I was hearing something else as her advocate. Loop back to ask questions.

Chapter 7 - Online Shopping - Check it out online first before buying online or otherwise

As I was trying to purchase medical accessories for my wife for use at home, I was lucky to have a friend from high school who ran a medical supply store. His staff helped me enormously in understanding my wife's needs and recommending the best equipment or accessories to purchase. But also, I learned from their questions to me, about my wife's condition and needs, about how to evaluate her equipment needs independently online and whether an intended purchase would work in the layout of our house.

I bought very few items online, as I did most of my purchases at my friend's medical supply store. But doing online research helped me enormously. Reading the postings of what people liked or disliked about a particular product helped me decide which particular piece of equipment I thought would work best for my wife in our house.

After I made an initial decision about a particular purchase, I would go to the medical supply store and ask the staff about the purchase. As they were becoming familiar with my wife's situation, they could offer their experienced insights into whether what I wanted to purchase was best. Another reason why I purchased from them was because they could get the item overnight and if it didn't work out, they would accept it back from me with no charge – they would put it in their stock for someone else.

A third reason why I didn't purchase online was that the larger items were generally medically prescribed by our doctors. As my wife was on Medicare, the store knew how to do the paperwork (and there was enough of it) and made it easy for me.

So, while for the most part, I have embraced the Internet and online shopping, there are times, such as this, that real human interaction still mattered.

Thank you Greg Ferraro, Jason and the staff of Robert Jacobson's Pharmacy for your friendship and professionalism. Thank you Fordham Prep for bringing Greg and me together.

Chapter 8 - Make LISTS - don't rely on your memory - it will fail you under stress

- Make a master list of things that need to be done, such as estate issues, funeral home, changing legal titles on houses, cars, other joint property, etc.
- Make a list of meaningful and necessary people to contact - family, friends, co-workers, bankers, lawyers, insurance agents, stock broker, pension and retirement plans managers
- Make daily lists of things to do that can actually be accomplished - it will help you feel better that you completed the daily task list
- Making daily lists will help you multi-task - multi-tasking is NOT doing everything at once, but doing many different things one at a time within the time allotted

Make a master list of things that need to be done, such as estate issues, funeral home, changing legal titles on houses, cars, other joint property, etc.

You might feel overwhelmed at this task, but don't think you have to do it all in one sitting. Start with a blank piece of paper and start jotting things down (or if you prefer to use an electronic journal). Don't worry yet about the order or sequence. When you can't think of anything else at the moment, stop and put the paper in your pocket and keep it handy with you.

As you go about your day, you will remember other things to add to the list. Pull out the piece of paper and add or modify it. If you do this often enough, you will soon need a new piece of paper as you will begin to see how to organize by category. You will go through many versions with additions and deletions.

If you have completed a task or item, make a check mark or something, but do not eliminate it from the next list you create – you want to remember that you have completed this task/item. Trust me, as the time progresses, and the stress and challenges increase, your memory will falter.

<u>Make a list of meaningful and necessary people to contact - family, friends, co-workers, bankers, lawyers, insurance agents, stock broker, pension and retirement plans managers</u>

This list may overlap with the master list, but this is more of a contact sheet than a "to do" list. Put the name and contact form – telephone, cell, email or regular mail, or any or all that will be needed.

Regarding family, friends and co-workers, you may want to set up a group email list and send out updates to the group on the patient's situation. If you wish for the recipients not to see each other's email addresses, put all the names into the "bcc" section as email addresses. This way, no recipient can see that another person also received the same email.

However, if you choose to start regular email updates, be prepared to: (1) respond individually to one or more recipients who will always want more information; (2) provide a regular update – otherwise people will think that your silence is bad news, even if nothing has happened and you just got sidetracked. So, think hard about starting any type of regular updates. (I decided not to start this as I knew I would be spending almost 50% of my day answering and following up on emails and phone calls – once I did it for one person, I would have to do it for everyone on the list.)

<u>Make daily lists of things to do that can actually be accomplished - it will help you feel better that you completed the daily task list</u>

There are a couple of reasons to make daily lists (which you can discard after completion or rollover outstanding items to the next daily list).

First, it helps to shrink down the enormity of the tasks before you to a manageable size. Don't put more than 5 or 6 items on the daily list. Also, expect that it will take twice as long as usual or estimated to accomplish any one task or the tasks collectively. Give yourself enough time, even if it appears more than ample. You will be surprised how quickly the day gets away from you.

Second, by being able to complete the daily list, it will give you a psychological sense of achievement – there will be many days when you will encounter frustration and despair and having something that can be accomplished is good for the soul.

Next to each item, put a number, starting with 1, to indicate a priority in which the tasks should be done each day. Generally, my daily list had either time sensitive tasks or tasks that can be arranged to minimize my travel time. When does the bank open and close so I have enough time to do banking activities? If I have to do outdoor work, does the weather forecast indicate the time of day that I need to accomplish an outdoor task? What sequence of chores or errands will be most efficient and how can I logically go from one place to the other? All these things I thought through having my first cup of coffee, preferably alone so that I was not distracted in thinking through my upcoming day.

In terms of dealing with banks and other institutions, as the customer service person either in person or on the phone does not usually deal with situations such as ours, assume you will need sufficient time to allow the customer service person(s) (you'll probably be transferred on the phone a few times) to deal with your questions.

Making daily lists will help you multi-task - multi-tasking is NOT doing everything at once, but doing many different things one at a time within the time allotted

The daily list will most likely be a mixture of different type of activities that require use of different parts of your brain or brawn. Being a good multi-tasker is to focus on the task at hand, do it and complete it. Don't be distracted by what is next on the list until you have completed the task at hand. If you have sequenced your day properly in the morning, you shouldn't have to worry about the next task until you are ready to deal with it (unless of course some event or emergency causes you to re-shuffle your schedule – WHICH WILL HAPPEN)

If your daily plan gets disrupted in a major way, then you need to remain calm and look at the list and ask yourself, "Must anything on this list be done today? Or can it wait till tomorrow?" Regardless of where the "must do" item is in the sequence of the list, push that up to number one and figure out how to do it. After that, play it by ear.

Chapter 9 - Enough Time to Do Daily Tasks

- Everything will take twice as long to get to or complete - this is OK - don't overload your daily task list

This is very important – I didn't realize how much more time it took to get simple tasks done, even if I had done them in the past.

So, I am repeating what I said in the previous chapter – GIVE YOURSELF ENOUGH TIME EACH DAY TO COMPLETE THE DAILY TASKS ON THE LIST.

Chapter 10 - Being an Athlete and Knowing When You're Hitting the Wall

- When do you "call a time out?" Or "take yourself out of the game"?

In looking back, one of the things that helped me greatly was my experience as an athlete (totally amateur – I never even lettered in high school).

You may start out strong, but as the game or competition wears on, you will wear down. At whatever sport, experienced athletes, over time, begin to recognize when they're getting tired – physically, mentally and emotionally. But sometimes they don't – that's why the baseball manager comes out on to the mound to relieve the pitcher who is losing effectiveness. But the pitcher is pumped up on adrenalin and always disputes that he has "lost it". If the manager then lets the pitcher continue against his better judgment, the rest usually will be history and disaster.

The caregiver must also give care to him or herself. If you break down, two people suffer – you and the patient. They say the best medicine is prevention. This is never more true than the case of caring for yourself.

In many sports (baseball, basketball, football (American)), you can stop the game and someone can call a time out, either a player or the coach/manager, when they sense that the momentum or trend of the game is going against them. The stoppage in play is intended for everyone to take a breather, re-group, re-think, collect oneself, etc.

How does this translate into being a caregiver?

First, as an athlete, do you know yourself and the limits of your physical and mental abilities - when you are at the top of your game and when you are not (i.e. tired, frustrated, injured)? Do you recognize when you are losing your edge as the game or contest progresses? What are the signs or symptoms of this?

If you do, then those signs or symptoms of your abilities declining during competition will also be the first signs to you as caregiver that you're "losing the edge".

Second, athletically, what have you done to restore your competitive edge? Maybe in some cases, as is the case for me when I play tennis, there is no alternative but to stop playing and rest. After 2 to 3 hours of tennis, I know I'm tired and a fresher, lesser rated player can beat me. I stopped playing, showered and went home.

Message: Stop being a caregiver for a necessary period of time. Do something that is not related to being a caregiver. How long this period is varies from person to person and it depends on the activity.

For me, one thing was tennis. During this period of my life, I continued to play tennis, even if I didn't feel 100%. But the difference was that my goal was to stay in some minimum level of physical shape and, use exercise to release my built-up stress. I DIDN'T TRY TO WIN EACH MATCH – I JUST WANTED THE EXERCISE AND THE STRESS RELEASE.

I also saw my friends and just chatted about various topics, anything but my wife's condition (I wouldn't avoid it if they asked, but I would not initiate that discussion). So, for a few hours on the weekends, I could take a mental break and try to keep in some level of physical shape.

Also, to take my mind away for a while, I would attend to business. During this time, I stopped working to take care of my wife full time. We were lucky that our financial resources were such that I could. I realize that this is not an option for many, probably most, people. But I still kept my finger in my business, but I involved myself in those aspects or situations that gave me satisfaction. As best I could, I avoided things about my business that annoyed or frustrated me, unless it was necessary.

(Again, for those who have to remain at work through this time period, I will not try to offer any suggestions. As I did not have to go through this experience, any comments I make would be pure speculation as to how I would have reacted or coped - my apologies.)

So, by totally taking my body and mind away from being a caregiver for a couple of hours per day allowed me to release my stress. I knew that I had to walk back into the frying pan, but it prevented me from burning out.

IT IS NOT SELFISH TO DO THIS. THE CAREGIVER IS THE SECOND PATIENT. PREVENTION IS THE BEST MEDICINE.

It is better that you are away from the patient and his/her needs for a relatively short period of time than to have you develop a chronic or acute physical or mental problem that forces you to be away for a longer period of time.

So figure out what activities will help you release your stress and don't feel selfish about them. It is just the opposite – you're helping both patients.

Chapter 11 - If Not an Athlete

- Did You Ever Work a "High Burn" Job - over 60 hours per week?

If you weren't an athlete on any level, then how do you pace yourself and know when you're reaching a critical stress point?

In my career, I have been a management consultant in a major firm where we regularly worked close to 60 hours a week, weekends and did a lot of traveling to clients. Sometimes the engagements were short and other times they were long. But often they were time sensitive with tight deadlines.

If you have been involved in these types of work situations, either as a lawyer, investment banker, or just someone who worked double shifts or two jobs, you probably have encountered the type of stress and fatigue of which I am writing about as a caregiver.

How and when did you recognize you were stressing out? How did you cope and release your stress while working under these conditions?

These are the past experiences that we must now use in the caregiver situation.

If the previous chapter and this chapter do not apply to your past experiences, I can only suggest that you pay close attention to your symptoms of fatigue, despair, frustration, fear, anything that you've never felt with as much intensity before. Also, if you have a close friend to whom you can ask to "watch your back" and warn you when they see you getting close to the edge, ask them to help you. You are NOT asking them to become the caregiver and take over your role – you're asking them to look out for you.

Chapter 12 - The Discipline to Sleep

- So That You Can Answer the Bell Every Morning - Eat Lightly, Sleep Deeply

Like a boxer, you have to walk back into the ring when the bell sounds for the next round. Every morning the bell sounds, figuratively and literally.

You have to get enough sleep to be refreshed and have the mental and physical strength to face and endure what the new day holds. And you will be severely pushed to the levels of your endurance.

For me, this was hard. I would lie in bed thinking about everything – did I forget to do something, thinking about the past and the future, EVERYTHING. Some nights I was too pumped up on adrenalin because something happened earlier and I had to go into "high gear" and react. Also, my wife would wake up in pain about every 3 hours and I would have to give her medication, or I would shift her physically to make her more comfortable.

One or two nights of this might be tolerable, but when it goes on for 7 days a week for an unknown period of time, you feel like you can't go on and will "lose it" very soon.

The only answer is to discipline yourself to sleep, take naps if possible during the day – even 10 minutes will help. The other tactic I used was to eat lunch as my main meal. This way, when I went to sleep, I was not sleeping on a full stomach. This allowed me to sleep more peacefully and deeply in between the periods of waking up to attend to my wife.

I use the word, "discipline", because it is too easy and natural to try to stay awake and keep thinking about everything that enters your mind. But you have to sleep; you have to force yourself to sleep – the bell rings again tomorrow and you MUST go back into the ring.

Endnote: Even now, a few months after my wife's passing and having sorted out most of the legal and administrative paperwork, I still find myself sitting up in bed awake, well into the night. I am still learning the <u>discipline</u> to sleep.

Chapter 13 - Down a Dark, Uncharted Road

- The Lost Summer - it's ok to feel down from time to time
- It hurts in the moment, but you WILL get through it - KEEP GOING
- How to keep playing even when the score says you're losing - what I learned from competitive sports
- When the race changes from a sprint to a marathon

The Lost Summer - it's ok to feel down from time to time

As my wife's situation progressively worsened from the end of winter through the summer, I look back and saw that it was a "Lost Summer", when I was scrambling and fighting a losing battle month to month. While it was weather-wise a very pleasant summer, it was all a blur to me and there were many nights when it all seemed so disheartening.

You do go through periods of frustration, despair, fear, uncertainty, anger, pain. It's okay – it's what you're supposed to feel.

It hurts in the moment, but you WILL get through it - KEEP GOING

But if I was able to get a reasonable night of sleep, I would have enough mental energy to keep going on. It hurts and there is emotional pain, but I had to keep going to give all the care I could for my wife. You have to believe that you will get through it. At that very moment, you may not know how you ever can, but you have to believe in yourself.

How to keep playing even when the score says you're losing - what I learned from competitive sports

Again, because of my competitive sports experience, I learned the discipline of not giving up hope even when you are losing. If you learn not to give up but take each day at a time and not let the whole situation overwhelm you, you have a chance to not losing control.

The good athletes learn how to handle the stress of the game and "keep their cool". This is what we must learn to do too.

When the race changes from a sprint to a marathon

There was one short period of time when my wife's situation seemed to stabilize and that there could be a longer period to her life, but with the existing level of incapacitation. This really took me back. While the medical professionals were saying that there was a short period of time remaining, there was a moment when it seemed she might become stable for a year or more, I had to stop and re-think my situation.

I had been doing the care giving at a very intense mental and physical level. If my wife were to be able to live closer to a year or more, I could not keep up this pace. I had to stop sprinting and start thinking about running a marathon. I will admit it scared and numbed me – the prospect of both of us living this way for that much longer a period of time.

While I started to try to adjust, trying to restore some of the personal parts of my life not related to my wife, her condition resumed its downward progression. To be honest, I don't know if I would have been able to adjust from "sprinting to running a marathon".

Endnote: I recently saw a newspaper article about injured war veterans returning from Iraq and the hardships for them and their spouses and families. These severely injured people had a prognosis of living years, maybe decades, in their horrible state. But I also thought of the spouses too. The soldiers and their spouses were easily twenty to twenty five years younger than I was. I couldn't imagine what their lives would be like going into the future. I am so sorry that I have no ideas nor anything I could say to them that I thought would be helpful.

Chapter 14 - Loving and Caring, BUT Annoying Friends

- Enough with the Food and Flowers Already (or whatever it is that annoys you)

There were many friends who offered and wanted to help. They wanted to send flowers or food.

From time to time in years past, when my wife was in the hospital for other reasons, invariably someone would send flowers. This annoyed both of us because it cluttered her hospital room and when she was discharged, we had to take all the flowers home with us.

So, we made a very conscious effort to tell all relatives and friends to NOT send flowers anywhere, not to the hospital, the rehab nursing home, our home. But, some people still insisted on sending flowers. We could be nothing but gracious, but it was just one more thing to deal with.

The other thing that annoyed me, personally, was food. People assumed that I needed to be fed properly and nutritiously. While it might be true that the male caregiver might be more likely to ignore proper eating habits, in my case (and all of our friends know this), I am the primary cook in our family. And I'm very aware of the value and need for good nutrition.

It wasn't that I didn't appreciate the kindness of our friends; I was running out of space in our refrigerator. In some ways, I was being forced to over eat just to keep the clutter out of the refrigerator and the freezer.

It seems that no matter what you tell some people, they will do whatever they want regardless.

For us, it was flowers and food. For some of you, it will be other gifts or acts of kindness or assistance that friends and family may want to give to you. I realize that family and friends are trying to be supportive and may feel very awkward as to how to be. They express that support in the most appropriate way they can. But it can be annoying because it is more trouble for you and it keeps you away from dealing with your job as a caregiver. After a while, I gave up trying to repeat the message.

At the end of the day, do the best you can to tell your friends and family about what NOT to do or send.

Chapter 15 - Coming to the End (for one patient)

- What does "Quality of Life" mean to both of you? It is not the same for everybody
- When to override the patient
- The vigil of the "last" phase
- The patient emotionally detaches from you - but don't be upset
- The last breath, my last thought

<u>What does "Quality of Life" mean to both of you? It is not the same for everybody</u>

The quality of life is an individual matter, as to when there is insufficient quality left. My wife was always a physically active and outdoor person. Although she liked to read, her greatest joys were to be outdoors – riding, gardening, and walking the dogs.

A few months before her passing, it became clear to both of us that she would not be able to enjoy these pleasures the way she would have liked. In the time period when we were still hopeful that her condition could be stabilized, there was hope of learning how to cope with some loss of these activities but retain some level of joy. If she had been able to, while her quality of life would have been diminished, I think we would have found some way to give her sufficient joy and quality to continue on.

It's my feeling that there is no moment of epiphany when either or both of you (the patient and caregiver) suddenly realize that the quality of life is totally gone. For me, I saw it slipping away, smaller and smaller, and finally realizing I couldn't see any joy in my wife's daily existence. By then, my wife was not able to cogently communicate with me and I realized that I was left making decisions for both of us.

When to override the patient

I wrote earlier in Chapter 4 about how the caregiver needed to progressively treat the patient more and more like a child in reverse. This was now becoming the case for us. In times when I sensed my wife was speaking or acting cogently, I would respect her wishes or accommodate her. But those times became less and less, and in fact, her responsiveness to me, as her caregiver, was less than her responsiveness to other people altogether.

You will have to make those decisions for the patient, even if you are not sure it's what he/she would have wanted. I live with that uncertainty, even to this day.

The patient emotionally detaches from you - but don't be upset

The home hospice nurse told me that it was known that some patients, knowing they are coming to the end, will stop reacting or interacting with the ones they most love. They have begun to detach themselves so that they would not feel sadness at leaving loved ones behind. It was clear to me that my wife would respond to the home health aide and to the nurse, but she was not responding to me. But the nurse did also say that my wife was capable of hearing or listening to me and others, but that she chose not to, or could not toward the end, respond. In fact, her hearing became possibly more acute as her brain was rechanneling somehow her remaining energy to those cognitive skills she still retained. (It seemed to me in retrospect that hearing is a passive function, whereas speaking or using the eyes requires active physical exertion, which may be one reason that hearing is one of the senses that remains working.) Eventually, she would also stop responding to them as well as she came to the end.

The vigil of the "last" phase

This was (and still is in some ways) the most difficult part for me. I was watching her literally die a little more every day and I was torn between not wanting to see her die, but yet hoping that she would be out of her misery as soon as possible. We are conditioned that life, in any form, under any situation, is preferable to dying. I don't know if I still believe that now. I knew she was alive, possibly capable to still hearing us and therefore having mental functions. But she could not communicate anymore to us – what was she thinking? Were there some last thoughts, words or instructions she wanted to say to me. Was she trying to hold on, or was she trying to let go?

My only solace is that the nurse who was now coming every day to visit confirmed to me that my wife seemed not to be in pain.

Prior to the last four weeks on home hospice, my wife would always be in pain and needed medication approximately every three hours, day or night. I would be the one to administer her medication (during the times she was home). But after she finally came home for the last time, her need for pain medicine suddenly decreased. Instead of every three hours, I was only administering to her the pain medication maybe three times per day. At first, I thought that maybe she was not able to communicate to me her pain, but the hospice nurse confirmed that my wife seemed not to be in pain, based on her experience.

I also asked the nurse how much longer my wife would hold out. The nurse replied that patients sometimes are waiting for someone or something to occur. Her mind was still functioning on some level.

<u>The last breath, my last thought</u>

One day, the hospice nurse, on her daily visit, came to us in the middle of her standard morning examination of my wife. She thought that before she proceeded further with her examination, which involved physically moving my wife around in bed, we might want to go and say our last words to my wife. (Her twin brother and sister-in-law were visiting me at the time.) I don't know what their reaction was, but I felt my heart stop for a second as I tried to gather myself calmly.

We went to see her, one by one. I went first and as I walked into our bedroom, I heard her brother cry silently as they waited for me.

I told her I loved her and recited the lyrics from a song I wrote for her almost thirty years ago, which she cherished very much. I hope she heard me.

She later passed away that day, some short time after the twelve o'clock siren sounded from the nearby firehouse, as it did every day. It is my belief that my wife chose to wait till after twelve noon to pass on. It occurs to me that she may have even lasted until the next day, but she may have given us her last act of love.

Her twin brother had driven up from Virginia and we were expecting a major hurricane to strike our area within two days. I believe that she could hear the conversations I had with her brother about when he would drive back. Clearly, he wanted to be with her at the end, but within two days, her brother would have been caught in the hurricane on the drive back. (The hurricane that hit the East Coast, in the New York area on August 27, 2011, was one of the largest hurricanes in recent memory.)

She waited until it was after twelve o'clock noontime in New York, as internationally, it was already the next day in Asia, August 26. That is the anniversary of my father's death. My wife and father then passed away on the same day.

She wanted her brother to miss the storm and go back a day earlier, but also wanted to spare me two days a year in which I would grieve for my loved ones.

She chose her time to go, thinking, loving and caring about us, even at the very end.

Endnote: I want to thank Elizabeth Darkey and Marcia Codner, the two home health aides who helped my wife and me on a daily basis. Also, I want to thank the people at Sloan Kettering Memorial Cancer Center, Northern Westchester Hospital, Somers Manor Nursing Home, the Lewisboro Volunteer Ambulance Corps, the Visiting Nurse Association of Hudson Valley, A&J Homecare and the Visiting Nurse Service of Westchester.

Chapter 16 - The Service and Arrangements - the easy "stuff" (the rest is more difficult)

- Wills, Health proxies, Living Wills, DNRs (Do Not Resuscitate)
- Making arrangements in a global environment - how to let faraway people grieve

<u>Wills, Health Proxies, Living Wills, DNRs (Do Not Resuscitate)</u>

If you have not gotten your wills, health proxies and living wills in place or made them current, I recommend that you do so immediately. You want to see as many matters resolved in a way that you and the patient want. Leaving these undone or not updated will leave you vulnerable to other people controlling your future – and possibly in a way against both your wishes.

The Do Not Resuscitate (DNR) instruction is an important one at the end. If you do not want emergency or medical care givers to try every last means to revive the patient, then this document relieves them of the legal liability of not doing so. But this is a decision you and the patient must make.

If the patient is hospitalized, ask the nurses / doctor to arrange for this PINK colored document to be implemented. If the patient is at home, have the home hospice agency coordinate the issuance of the DNR.

The home hospice will tell you, and I repeat what they said to me – if there is an emergency that happens at home, do NOT call 911 or the local medical emergency number. Call the home hospice on their 24-hour line. They will make the necessary calls. The reason is that if you call 911 or the local ambulance agency directly, when they show up at your home, they will be required to take all necessary actions, even if you have a DNR. They are legally bound to ignore the DNR.

So, call the home hospice number first and follow their instructions.

Making arrangements in a global environment - how to let faraway people grieve

We have several close friends who live overseas or faraway. Several of them could not come to any memorial service that I could have arranged.

So, at the service, I hired a videographer to film the proceedings, film the speakers. Then, a separate video clip was made of each person who spoke. I received the DVD with all of them and I posted them on my YouTube account. I sent the links to all the people who could not attend so that they could at least watch and hear others. (As some of you know, you can set the parameters of each video posted on YouTube so that only people to whom you have sent the link can view the video. This way you can keep it private.)

Chapter 17 - Coming to the New Beginning (for the "other" patient)

- How does one move on?

This is an incomplete chapter, maybe to be finished in another book.

I don't want to describe here all of my feelings and emotions because I haven't sorted them out yet to make sense of them for myself to try to explain to anyone else.

Cleaning out the closets, beginning to discard clothing, disbursing her personal valuables to nieces and nephews and other physical activities seemed necessary for me to start moving on.

I wrote and published a second book of poems, all written in the last several months of my wife's illness. This was part of my emotional and psychological therapy. (It is available through Amazon in Kindle and paperback. The title is Dark Passage – Travels on the Inner Road II.)

This book was also written as part of that process, looking for something good, a greater good, to come from something that hurt – making better lemonade.

To be continued…

www.ingramcontent.com/pod-product-compliance
Lightning Source LLC
Chambersburg PA
CBHW071548170526
45166CB00004B/1583